Urban *Goddess* Mama-to-Be

A Simple Guide to a Magical Pregnancy

Melania Tolan

Copyright © 2014 by **Melania Tolan**

All rights reserved. No part of this publication may be reproduced, distributed, or transmitted in any form or by any means, without prior written permission.

Melania Tolan
PO BOX 16222
PORTLAND, OR 97216
www.melaniatolan.com

Publisher's Note: The author acknowledges the copyrighted or trademarked status and the trademark owners of any workmark mentioned in the work of nonfiction.

The author does not dispense medical advice. Please consult your medical provider for treatment and advice.

Cover Design by Christy Caughie at http://gildedheartdesign.com

Cover photography by Eric Hudson

Cover Model: Susan Malone

Book Layout © 2014 BookDesignTemplates.com

Urban Goddess Mama-to-Be/ Melania Tolan. -- 1st ed.
ISBN 978-0-9904007-3-8

To my Wise Women sisters

A grand adventure is about to begin.
—WINNIE THE POOH

CONTENTS

First Trimester 1
   CHOOSING A PROVIDER 2
   NUTRITION 7
   RECIPES 13
   EXERCISE 15
   MORNING SICKNESS 21
   ADVICE & THE OPINIONS OF OTHERS 23
Second Trimester 27
   MEDITATION & MINDFULNESS 28
   LOVE YOUR BODY 30
   SELF-CARE 32
   CHILDBIRTH CLASSES 37
   MATERNITY CLOTHES 39
   PREPARING YOUR HOME 41
Third Trimester 45
   DOULA 48
   FINDING A PEDIATRICIAN 49
   PREPARING YOURSELF 51
   BIRTH PLAN 53
   BREASTFEEDING 54
   HOSPITAL/BIRTH BAG 57
   POSTPARTUM DEPRESSION 59
   THE BLESSING WAY 61
New Beginnings 73

PREFACE

Dear Mama-To-Be,

I wanted to write the book I wish I had when I was pregnant: short, sweet, and to the point. Every book I looked at was at least 300 pages or more, and many of them read like textbooks. Already overwhelmed with the fact I was pregnant, I paged through them, only to set them down and never look at them again. Disappointed, I relied extensively on the internet for advice. My midwife provided some resources, but all I wanted was a brief guide covering the basic topics.

A year after our daughter arrived, I completed a short memoir, *Urban Goddess Mama*, about my battle with postpartum depression. In the process of publishing that book, I realized my next project should be for the Mama-to-be, the book that I wished I had a year before. Over the next six months I wrote down different topics that had been of interest for me that I wished I'd had more information on during my pregnancy. Thus *Urban Goddess Mama-to-Be* was conceived.

It is my greatest desire that you not only find this book helpful in your journey, as you transition from maiden to mother and that you gain the necessary knowledge to enhance your experience during these magical months, but that it also helps you prepare for the postpartum period. Pregnancy is an enchanting time of transformation, however, when the baby arrives, things will drastically change. That doesn't mean the magic has to end after childbirth, preparing for the grand baby debut is vital to a smooth transition.

This book is written for the expecting first time mama and is split into three parts to mirror the three trimesters. Each part is then subdivided into specific topics which pertain to that period of pregnancy. However, each subject may be applicable at any time during pregnancy. This is a simple guide, without too much detail, because these topics have been covered in much deeper depth through countless articles and books. My goal is simply to introduce each concept, and if the topic resonates with you, you can explore additional information. I have added links to online resources at the end of each section and a few magical goddess tips.

Be sure you check in with your healthcare provider before applying any of the concepts in this book, as each person's body and situation is unique. I wish you the very best on your amazing journey into motherhood. Enjoy this magical time.

Much love to you, Mama-to-be,

Melania Tolan

PART ONE

First Trimester

You just found out you're expecting. Maybe this is a planned pregnancy or perhaps it is completely unexpected. Whatever your situation, you probably have a whirlwind of emotions and thoughts coursing through you like an angry hurricane. There are so many things to think about.

Where will the baby fit in our home and lives? Can I work full-time after the baby arrives, or even work at all? What about that vacation I wanted to take with my partner? Will I be able to do it now that I'm pregnant? Will "it" be a girl or a boy? Where am I going to deliver this new little person growing inside me? Will I go with a typical hospital birth or try a natural home birth? What can I eat? Can I continue my exercise routine? And so on and so forth.

Then there are those pesky little things called hormones. I would feel great one moment, and then my cat came over to nuzzle me with his wet nose, and I burst into tears. I was uncertain if the water-works were joyous or sad, but there they were. Hello, emotional roller coaster! My poor husband would pat my knee or massage my shoulders trying to be supportive, but I'm sure my moodiness got to him too. Who knew that one tiny sperm and egg coming together could cause such disruption in a person's life? As you begin this journey, keep in mind that your pregnancy is very unique, while there are certain benchmarks as to what you should be experiencing at each stage of gestation, sometimes your "normal" may be someone else's abnormal, and vice-versa. This is one of the reasons that it's important to establish prenatal care and get all the initial exams and tests done promptly.

CHOOSING A PROVIDER

When I found out I was pregnant, I sat on the couch for the entire four-day weekend I had off, and played the game Bejeweled on my phone when I wasn't sleeping or getting something to eat. Thoughts swirled through my brain as I contemplated how the positive pregnancy test I had taken the Friday before had changed everything. All the goals and timelines I had previously established for my writing, career, and financial situation had suddenly changed. What I had once thought was so important didn't matter now, and things I had never considered before became a vital part of my life.

I thought about all the books I had wanted to write before I started a family. Was it possible to get them done before the baby was born? I spent hours crunching numbers, figuring out how much money we needed to save so I could take the full length of my allotted maternity leave. Where would we put the baby and all of the baby stuff? We lived in a two-bedroom, 850-square-feet apartment. Space was at a premium.

Round and round my brain went, trying to figure out just how this change would affect our lives, continuing through most of my pregnancy. One of my immediate concerns was deciding what route to take as far as medical care, especially because I was already leaning toward natural childbirth (no medical interventions.

I went into my OB-GYN's office during one of my lunch breaks and scheduled an appointment with her. She booked out fast and I wanted to get in as soon as possible. I was also considering going with the midwives at the hospital I worked for. I'd watched The Business of Being Born, and I knew I wanted to have a natural birth, maybe even a home birth. My first gut reaction was to go see the doctor I trusted the most.

When I scheduled my appointment, I had a mixture of relief and anxiety with a bit of guilt. If I really wanted a natural birth, why was I scheduling my appointments with a medical doctor? This bothered me enough to also start looking for a midwife since my first appointment wouldn't be for another month. I looked into the midwives through the hospital, as well as several independent birthing centers.

One of the centers a friend suggested after her own positive experience appealed to me. I met with the midwife my friend had seen and liked her instantly. The only thing that bothered me was she'd never had any children of her own. But this time I pushed past the anxious feeling in my gut because I really liked her.

My appointment with the original OB was rescheduled because she had an emergency procedure to perform, and I ended up seeing her partner, who I also trusted. He'd delivered my cousin's baby and also performed a surgery on my best friend. He cleared me for a natural birth, at home if I chose, and I transferred my prenatal care to the midwife.

Throughout the pregnancy, the midwife and her two assistants gave me fantastic care. Unfortunately, as I got closer to my delivery date, I became more and more anxious about my choice of childbirth options and this time I couldn't shake the feeling. When I did verbalize my feelings at an appointment, I was told this was totally normal, and that all expectant mothers feel this before the "big day." The anxiety began to interfere with my ability to sleep the closer I got to the end of the forty weeks. I kept thinking I should have stayed with the OB clinic I had originally gone to and have a hospital birth. I could still try for a natural birth in the hospital. I felt safer there for some reason, but part of me dismissed this as cultural fears.

"Stop being such a chicken, Melania," I told myself every time these worries crept up. "Thousands of women deliver babies every day without the help of drugs or a physician."

When I finally went into labor, things didn't turn out the way I had planned, and I ended up in the hospital after laboring for over twelve hours between home and the birthing center. The moment the assistant midwife wheeled me in the hospital, every cell of my body relaxed and I knew this is where I should have been the whole time. All the nurses and the hospital midwives who took over my care had children of their own. They had been there, done that. They knew exactly what I was going through.

My advice to new moms is to look deeply and honestly into your heart and make the choice that feels right to you. Don't let anyone tell you "the natural" or "the hospital" way is the only "right" way. You should only do what feels right to you. If a home birth resonates with you then go for it. Many women have had magical home births. If the hospital setting feels more in line with what you want, then find the provider and hospital that matches your intentions and desires. There is no right or wrong way. Things don't always go according to plan, especially with regard to childbirth. Shit happens, as the phrase goes, but if you are in the environment you feel most comfortable in, and supported by people who match your values, no matter what occurs, you know you made the right decision. Trust your intuition.

Ask yourself what is it that you want? What is important to you? Be honest and don't hold back. Write the answers down in a journal. Write your fears down too. Look at each answer and check within yourself. Go through each scenario and take note of how your body reacts.

If you still feel confused as to what you should do, schedule appointments with all the providers you are considering, tour birthing centers and hospitals, talk to friends and family about their experiences and/or recommendations, go online and research. With each visit, check in with yourself and see how you feel or your body responds. Take your time in making the decision. Do your research.

Obviously, if you are having any medical issues, you need to seek care immediately, but otherwise there isn't any rush. While you wait for your initial appointment, make sure you start taking a good prenatal vitamin. I liked Rainbow brand prenatal vitamins, because they use natural sources for the vitamins, and they donate a percentage of the profits to provide vitamins to people in developing countries. We'll cover more about that in the Nutrition section.

Magical Goddess Tip:

Most importantly, trust your body. If you feel something is off, or need peace of mind knowing everything is okay, make sure to voice your concern to whomever you are seeing.

Typically they book the initial appointment no earlier than seven to eight weeks, unless you have been receiving fertility care, considered high risk, or are experiencing extreme nausea and vomiting from "morning sickness." Do not be afraid talk about your fears. If this is your first pregnancy, anxiety and apprehension are normal. That is why it's important to trust your gut and listen to what your body is telling you.

No matter which route you choose to go with for prenatal care and childbirth, if things don't go according to plan, it is very common for mothers to second-guess their decisions. I know I did so many times. Part of me wishes I'd gone with my original OB, but I also wonder, if I'd done that, would I always wonder what a natural water birth at the birthing center would have been like? The answer is maybe, but I'm not going to waste any more time thinking of what I should or shouldn't have done. The past is done. I know for the future, if we choose to have baby 2.0, we'll be going to the hospital that also offers water birth, with the midwives at my OB's clinic.

Shannon Brown of Growing Slower has a great checklist of questions to ask your provider once you find one:
http://www.growingslower.com/2013/10/obstetrician-midwife-interview-questions.html

NUTRITION

You may have noticed that your appetite has grown significantly over the last few weeks. Growing a human takes a lot of energy, so getting the proper nutrition is super important. If you've already established care with a medical provider, they may have already addressed the importance of getting enough protein. Proteins provide the essential amino acids needed for fetal development.

If you eat meat, this is easy to facilitate, but if you are a vegetarian like me, getting the necessary protein can seem tricky. However finding good protein sources is not as complicated as it seems. Below is a list of plant-based ingredients that are rich in protein.

1. **Vegetables** – (the foundation for all diets)
    - 1 avocado - 10 grams
    - 1 cup boiled peas - 9 grams
    - 1 cup broccoli - 5 grams
    - 1 cup spinach - 5 grams
    - 2 cups cooked kale - 5 grams
    - 1 cup cooked sweet potato - 5 grams

2. **Legumes** – (specifically lentils and beans, the foundation of many diets for centuries)
    - 1 cup soybeans - 28 grams
    - For soybean based products:
        - 1 cup tempeh - 30 grams

- o 1 cup tofu - 22 grams
- 1 cup lentils - 18 grams
- 1 cup refried beans - 15.5 grams
- 1 cup garbanzo beans (and hummus) - 14.5 grams
- 1 cup pinto, kidney, black beans - 13-15 grams
- 1 ounce peanuts - 6.5 grams

3. **Nuts and Seeds** – (a staple in most vegetarian and vegan diets)
- 1 ounce sesame seeds - 6.5 grams; 3 tablespoons of tahini - 8 grams
- 1 ounce pistachios - 5.8 grams
- 1/4 cup (2 ounces) walnuts - 5 grams
- 1 ounce cashews - 4.4 grams
- 2 tablespoons almonds - 4 grams
- Nut butters - peanut butter, almond butter, cashew butter - 2 tablespoons has about 8 grams of protein

4. **Non-dairy milk** – (Soy, almond, ancient grain) - 1 cup 7-9 grams of protein

5. **Grains** – (Ancient grains, sprouted grains, multi-grains)
- Quinoa 1 cup - 9 grams
- Amaranth, bulgur, brown rice, wheat germ, oat bran are other grains with a high protein content
- Seitan, (or flavored wheat gluten) - approx. 52 grams per cup, but it may not be a good idea if you have wheat sensitivity
- Oatmeal 1 cup - 6 grams
- Sprouted grain bread products – (buns, tortillas, bread) 7-10 grams

6. **Convenience foods**: There are vegan protein powders and bars to fill in the gaps on the go. Hemp - 30 grams of hemp powder in your smoothie gives you 11 grams of protein.

7. **Supplements** - spirulina and chlorella are often used by vegetarians and vegans for their rich nutrient content, and protein content.
(http://www.naturalnews.com)

Here are examples of how I got my daily recommended servings of protein.

Breakfast:
20 oz. smoothie with 15 grams of protein powder, kale, banana, soy milk (5 grams of protein), 1 cup of Greek yogurt (5 grams of protein), fresh berries or mangos (25 grams total)
Or
2 slices of whole grain gluten-free waffles (10 grams of protein, recipe at end of the section), 2 tablespoons of any nut butter (5 grams of protein), 2 pieces of fresh fruit, and a glass of soy milk (5 grams of protein) (20 grams total)

Morning snack:
1 hard-boiled egg sliced on whole grain bread toast with a slice of cheese (10 grams total)
Or 2 slices of cheese and an apple (10 grams total)

Lunch:
Fresh salad with 1 cup of garbanzo, black, or white beans (10 grams protein), handful of nuts & seeds (3-5 grams of protein) (15 grams total)

Or
Quinoa salad with beans & fresh veggies (15 grams total)
Or
Mediterranean wrap with hummus, feta cheese, tzatziki sauce, and falafels (10-15 grams of protein)

Afternoon Snack:
Protein bar (10 grams of protein, Luna or Lara bars are my favorite)
Or
1 cup of berries with a cup of yogurt (5-7 grams of protein)
Or
Veggie sticks with a ½ cup of hummus (5-7 grams of protein)

Dinner:
Pasta with shredded cheese (5-7 grams of protein)
Or
Beans and rice with steamed veggies and shredded cheese (10 grams of protein)
Or
Mac and cheese with veggies (5-7 grams of protein)

Bedtime snack:
1 banana with a cup of warm soy milk (5 grams of protein)
Or
1/3 cup of nuts (5 grams)
Or
1 slice of cheese with wholegrain crackers (5 grams of protein)

The options listed above are just a few ideas of how to get your daily servings of protein. I found if I could get the highest amount of protein in the first part of my day, I didn't have to worry if I was getting enough, and I felt energized throughout my day.

My midwife recommended 65 grams of protein per day. I couldn't stomach that much protein. For me, 50-55 grams felt right. I made this known to her and everything worked out okay. Listen to your body. Maybe you need more than 65 grams, or less, but make sure you discuss this with your provider and get a plan in place that matches your needs.

Omega acids

Omegas 3 and 6 are vital to fetal development. Fish is rich in omegas, but during pregnancy you should limit your intake of fish due to mercury content. I usually don't eat meat, but when I was about three-months pregnant I started craving fish. A girlfriend mentioned Wild Planet Canned Tuna (www.wildplanetfoods.com) that is low in mercury because the tuna fish is caught when they are smaller so they haven't had enough time to absorb the metal. I made myself a tuna salad every other week and ate it over two or three meals during the course of the week.

My husband also discovered a great plant-based source of omegas called Udo's Choice oil, which contains a blend of flaxseed, sesame, sunflower, and other oils. I wasn't particularly fond of the taste however, so I would mix it into different foods, like my morning protein smoothie or mix a tablespoon of the oil in a cup of ice cream with a handful of nuts. Walnuts are also an excellent source of omega, and can be added to cereal or salads.

Shortly after my daughter's first birthday, I discovered The Honest Company DHA/Omega-3 gel caps. They are the first omega/fish oil supplements I've found that didn't have the fishy aftertaste or upset my stomach. The oil is harvested from small fish to decrease mercury exposure. I wish I'd had them during my pregnancy.

Prenatal Vitamins
There are many brands out there, so whichever one you choose, make sure it has at least 400 mcg folic acid, as well as calcium, iron, and B vitamins. Check with your provider for suggestions on which minerals you need. Each body is different and requires different vitamins. Again, Rainbow brand worked really well for me. I took The Honest Company prenatal vitamins postpartum and I liked them too.

Eating balanced meals and snacks is so important to gain the proper nutrition. Make sure you include an item from each food group in every meal.

Magical Goddess Tip:
Eat a full spectrum of colors when it comes to vegetables and fruit to ensure you are getting all the nutrients your body needs.

Hydration
Mamas-to-be need to drink lots of water. According to the Institute of Medicine, pregnant women should drink about 10 8oz. cups of water (http://www.mayoclinic.org/healthy-

living/nutrition-and-healthy-eating/in-depth/water/art-20044256?pg=2). Make sure you get plenty of electrolytes too. An excellent natural source is coconut water. I used to drink a can a day. Avoid any sugar-based electrolyte drinks that are filled with artificial flavors and dyes.

For more information on prenatal nutrition, check out the following websites:

American Pregnancy
http://americanpregnancy.org/pregnancyhealth/pregnancynutrition.html

The Cleveland Clinic
http://my.clevelandclinic.org/healthy_living/pregnancy/hic_nutrition_during_pregnancy_for_vegetarians.aspx

Veg Kitchen
http://www.vegkitchen.com/nutrition/vegetarian-pregnancy/

RECIPES

Garbanzo-Oat Waffles (Gluten Free)
(Originally from Recipes Goodness Pure & Simple by Lloyce Olson & Yolanda Leamon, printed by Morris Press, Kearney, NE)

2¼ c. water

1½ c. rolled oats
1 c. soaked garbanzos (½ cup dry)
2 dates
2 tbsp. raw sunflower seeds
2 tsp. vanilla
½ teaspoon salt

Preheat waffle iron. Blend all the ingredients together. Coat waffle iron with a non-stick spray. Bake in hot waffle iron for 8-10 minutes. Every waffle iron is a little different in the time required and serving sizes may vary.

I like to add a couple of teaspoons of cinnamon or a half cup of almond meal. These waffles are delicious and are packed with protein.

Black Bean Burgers (from www.allrecipes.com)
1 (16 oz) can black beans, drained and rinsed
½ green bell pepper, cut into 2-inch pieces
½ onion, cut into wedges
3 cloves garlic, peeled
1 egg
1 tbsp. chili powder
1 tbsp. cumin (I like to put in 2 for extra flavor)
1 tsp. Thai chili sauce or hot sauce
½ c. bread crumbs

If grilling, preheat an outdoor grill for high heat and lightly oil a sheet of aluminum foil. If baking, preheat oven to 375 degrees F (190 degrees C) and lightly oil a baking sheet.

In a medium bowl, mash black beans with a fork until thick and pasty.

In a food processor, finely chop bell pepper, onion, and garlic. Stir into mashed beans. In a small bowl, stir together egg, chili powder, cumin, and chili sauce.

Stir the egg mixture into the mashed beans. Mix in bread crumbs until the mixture is sticky and holds together. Divide mixture into four patties.

If grilling, place patties on foil and grill about 8 minutes on each side. If baking, place patties on baking sheet and bake about 10 minutes on each side.

Pineapple Tofu Yogurt Smoothie
1 container of tofu (I prefer the Mori Nu Silk soft tofu)
1 can of pineapple (crushed or chunks)
1 c. of shredded coconut
(Optional) 1 cup frozen bananas or mangos

Blend until smooth. You can add some coconut milk to make into smoothie consistency.

EXERCISE

When I found out I was pregnant, the first concern I had was my physical fitness level so I joined the gym the following week. The only problem was I hated working out. After some online research on exercise for pregnancy, I discovered that swimming was one of the best exercises for pregnant women. I love swimming so I choose a gym with a nice low-chlorine saline pool to avoid as many chemicals as possible. The less chlorine the better.

I also went to a prenatal yoga class but soon became too tired to endure an entire hour-long class. Swimming and half-hour walks at lunch became my regular forms of exercise. Because of morning sickness, I could only do 20-30 minutes at a time. My daily 20-minute swim actually gave me the energy I needed to get through my 10-hour shift and help to decrease my nausea significantly.

However, when I started feeling better, I got lazy and stopped going to the gym. My fitness level declined soon after as did my energy level.

During my third trimester I started swimming again and doing a 25-minute yoga video I found on YouTube, but still I didn't push myself past the half-hour mark. While doing any exercise was good, I didn't increase my level of fitness and stamina needed for a long delivery. In the end, this may have made my recovery take longer than usual.

I didn't practice Kegel exercises either, which also affected my recovery post-birth. Therefore I cannot stress enough the importance of exercise during pregnancy, especially Kegels, which help strengthen the pelvic floor muscles you'll use to push the baby out. While having strong pelvic muscles is imperative, knowing how to fully relax them to let the baby through is equally vital. This is something I unfortunately learned after I gave birth.

Four months after my daughter was born, I started pelvic physical therapy due to intense pelvic floor pain and scar tissue in my perineal area from the third-degree tear I experienced during childbirth. During the third session of pelvic PT, my therapist identified the issue. I couldn't relax my pelvic floor which caused the muscles to spasm, resulting in pain. She also informed me that what I thought was "pushing" was actually the opposite; I was holding everything in. No wonder I'd had a hard time getting the baby out.

Part of this issue was poor childbirth education. I'd chosen a midwifery clinic for natural childbirth, and the midwives encouraged me to trust my body, assuring me that I'd know what to do when the time came. Unfortunately I didn't know what my body should be doing, and held everything inside instead of allowing my body to open up and release the baby. A class on basics of childbirth may have been helpful for me and we'll talk more about childbirth classes in the next chapter.

Before starting any form of exercise, make sure you get approval from your healthcare provider, and ensure that you don't have any risks which may affect your pregnancy. If you've been regularly working out prior to pregnancy, then you'll probably be okay to keep doing so, but may need to modify your current routine and should check with your provider anyway.

For those of you who haven't been exercising regularly prior to pregnancy, don't worry. You can build up your physical fitness over the course of your pregnancy. Here are some tips for starting an effective exercise program:

- Start small. Don't overdo it.
- Find an exercise buddy, someone who can motivate you and keep you on track.
- Make sure to diversify your routine. Doing the same walking course or class can get boring quick-

ly. Changing your program helps keep you motivated.
- Get a portable music device (such as an iPod or MP3 player) with headphones to load your favorite tunes or power music onto.
- Make sure you take a day of rest once or twice a week to allow your body to recover.
- Mix different types of exercises. If you do cardio one day, work with weights or cross-training the next day. Make sure by the end of the week you've targeted all of the muscle groups of the body.
- Don't forget to drink lots of water during and after you workout. Coconut water contains electrolytes and is perfect for post exercise hydration.
- Stretch, stretch, stretch! Drinking plenty of water and stretching before and after a workout helps flush out the lactic acid from the muscles which decreases soreness. Especially stretch your leg muscles including the hip flexors. Having flexible inner leg muscles helps when those tissues stretch during birth and can reduce the risk of tearing.

Types of exercises:
- **Walking**. For those of you looking to keep things simple, just start by walking for 15 minutes a day for the first week, 20 minutes the second week, and 30 the following week. When you reach a half-hour a day, 4-5 days a week, try increasing your speed, or add hills or stairs, to your routine. As you start challenging yourself, make sure that you don't overheat or push yourself too hard. A

great way to know if you are overdoing it is to check with your breath. You should be able to hold a conversation as you are exercising.
- **Squats.** It is super important to build those leg muscles. You'll rely on them when it comes time to push your baby out during delivery. Squatting is actually a common birthing position, because you've got gravity working with you. It's important to have strong legs muscles to maintain a squatting position during delivery. Start with 3 sets of 5-10 squats per day and slowly increase to 12-15 over a course of a week. If 10 seems too easy, start at 15 or do 2-3 extra sets.
- **Take a prenatal yoga class.** I so wish I had done yoga regularly during my pregnancy. I truly believe it would have made a world of difference during labor. Yoga not only tones your muscles, it also adds flexibility and teaches you to breathe; all of which are essential during labor and delivery. If you can't afford to attend a regular class, visit your local library, as they have lots of videos you can borrow for free.
- **Swimming.** This was my favorite form of exercise because I never felt like I was working out when I got in the pool. I also loved being in the water. The fact that swimming targets all the major muscle groups and provides cardio only made me love it more. I wish I would have allowed myself more time in the pool, because I always felt great after a good 30-40 minute swim. Being in the water also kept my body from overheating. In my third tri-

mester, I looked forward to getting in the water because the buoyancy relieved the growing belly weight. I loved floating on my back at the end of my swim and letting the water just hold me. I felt my muscles relax and even the baby. Those moments go down as the most magical during my pregnancy.

When you look for a class or video, make sure it contains squats, Kegel exercises, and relaxation techniques. Attending a fitness class was hard for me. Because of my work hours, the classes I wanted to attend usually occurred while I was at work or not at a convenient time. Gaiam, a company that provides fitness products and media, has dozens of excellent prenatal yoga videos, which I utilized. The problem for me was I didn't have the motivation to do them regularly. This is when a workout buddy plays an essential role. They don't have to be pregnant and they can still benefit from the yoga video.

Magical Goddess Tip:

Your partner or spouse can participate with you. It's a great way to bond and make them feel included in the pregnancy experience.

Check out Gaiam TV for streaming prenatal yoga videos. My favorite was the Radiant Pregnancy series. www.gaiamtv.com

MORNING SICKNESS

A week after I found out I was pregnant, I thought, "This isn't too bad." The following week, I woke up in the middle of the night feeling like I'd been sleeping on a boat in high seas, and the topsy-turvy sensation in my stomach lasted all day. Not once did I vomit; which actually made the nausea that much worse since I couldn't find relief.

I tried every suggestion I could find: eating saltines, drinking ginger ale, avoiding fried foods, drinking peppermint tea, and eating smaller, more frequent meals, etc. Some of these remedies helped; most didn't. After some online research, I discovered that exercise can also help with nausea, but I'd been far too sick to go to the gym.

One morning I forced myself to get up and go swim. I was skeptical about the being in a pool would be helpful with the seasick feeling I had, but after a few minutes of gentle movement through the water, I started to feel rejuvenated and less nauseous. At the end of my 20-minute swim, the nausea was almost gone and I felt more energized than I had the past few days. This motivated me to swim every morning throughout the first trimester. While the exercise didn't take the morning sickness away completely, I felt that moving my body did help bring the nausea to a bearable level.

At eight weeks, my husband and I celebrated our eighth wedding anniversary. This was going to be our last vacation together before the baby arrived, a babymoon if you will, and we planned a four-day trip to Victoria, British Columbia, traveling via train to Seattle and then by ferry to the island, without a thought about morning sickness. As our mini-holiday approached, I got nervous, thinking that we should have driven to Port Angeles, Washington, to take the shorter ferry from there.

My midwife suggested acupressure wrist-bands and ginger gum. Not once did I get seasick on the trip, using the bands while on the train and boat. I chewed the ginger gum at the beginning of the boat ride and that helped too. In fact, I chewed a piece every morning on the trip.

After we returned from our vacation, my cousin gave me an awesome tip. She told me that she used to put fresh slices of ginger into her water bottle and drink that all day, and in the evening, she'd put in fresh slices for nighttime drinking. I started doing this and the last bit of my nausea disappeared.

Everyone's body is different. Sometimes prenatal vitamins make the nausea worse, and ff that's the case, take them at night right before bed. Some women have seemingly done everything mentioned above without relief, or were so sick they couldn't even get out of bed. If you are one of those unfortunate souls, make sure you talk to your provider to develop a plan. Not being able to keep anything down can cause negative effects on your health and that of the baby, especially at this early stage of pregnancy.

Magical Goddess Tip:

Honor your body and the growing life within you
by taking time to rest.

For more tips on prenatal remedies check out these sites:
Mind Body Green

http://www.mindbodygreen.com/0-9602/30-natural-remedies-for-morning-sickness.html

Mayo Clinic
http://www.mayoclinic.org/diseases-conditions/morning-sickness/basics/definition/con-20033445

Pregnant Chicken
http://www.pregnantchicken.com/pregnant-chicken-blog/2010/9/29/15-morning-sickness-remedies.html

ADVICE & THE OPINIONS OF OTHERS

Nothing brings out people's opinions like a pregnant woman. Everyone from the old lady in the grocery line to the receptionist at your OB's office and the department store clerk will offer you some nugget of information regarding pregnancy, whether they have experienced pregnancy or not.

Your family and friends will offer advice and tell you all kinds of stories of their pregnancies. What they ate, how they slept, what kind of cravings they had, and what type of clothing they wore.

Most of the time, people are just excited to see a pregnant woman, and their way to connect is to share whatever experience they've had. Or in the case of your family and friends, they're so thrilled about you being pregnant that they have to share everything to "help" you.

However, as good as everyone's intentions may be, all this advice can be overwhelming. Many times, opinions are based on a period of time when circumstances and family dynamics were much different than they are now. What doctors used to recommend before is often now considered contraindicative. If your family or friends are constantly hounding you about what you should and shouldn't be doing, now is the time to establish healthy boundaries with your loved ones. Don't be afraid to say no or that you'd prefer they not share so much information because you're feeling overwhelmed by everything. If you mention that you're feeling stressed, people tend to understand and back away. Nobody wants to stress an expecting mama.

My mother is an amazing, brilliant physician who specializes in natural medicine, and basically is a walking encyclopedia for holistic health. When I finally told her I was pregnant, she had all kinds of ideas to share. Some were helpful, while others seemed like old-school myths, like concerns about indoor cats. She is still convinced to this day that indoor felines are a danger to one's health (pregnant or not). In her opinion, cats are especially hazardous to babies. She kept telling me what she'd heard and read about cats killing babies. I'd heard this before too, so I did some research online. It turns out there is only one documented instance of a cat causing the death of an infant. The coroner's report, however, states the baby didn't die of asphyxiation (from the cat) but of SIDS. I shared this with my mother, but it did little to change her opinion.

Instead, she began telling me of rare diseases that cats carry and can transmit to humans. While this is partially true, for example, a pregnant woman shouldn't touch or clean a kitty litter box because they could get toxoplasmosis, most diseases that indoor pets could have cannot be transmitted to humans. In fact, I found the opposite to be true, finding several studies done in Europe indicating that children growing up in homes with pets have better immune systems and less allergies, colds, ear infections, and asthma (http://healthland.time.com/2012/07/09/study-why-dogs-and-cats-make-babies-healthier/). I shared this information with her, but this still didn't stop her from constantly suggesting we get rid of our two indoor cats. I finally put my foot down and gently tell her we knew what was best for our family.

Establishing healthy boundaries is vital to a mama's sanity and also important when the baby arrives. Give yourself permission to be firm.

The Art of Extreme Self-care by Cheryl Richardson has a great chapter about establishing healthy boundaries and not letting people mow you over with well-intentioned but superfluous advice.

PART TWO

Second Trimester

I will never forget the feeling of reaching the end of the first trimester. I could breathe easier because the risk of miscarriage had gone down significantly and I could finally share the good news. Moving into the next trimester also meant less morning sickness and an increase in energy.

I started all kinds of projects around the house to prepare for the arrival of my little angel and even did a little traveling too.

The part I didn't care for much was that my baby bump wasn't quite showing but all my clothes no longer fit. For a while it just looked like I was gaining weight and by twelve weeks, I broke down and went maternity clothes shopping.

The second trimester was the best time in my pregnancy because I wasn't big yet but had all the benefits of being pregnant (larges breasts, glowing skin, amazing hair, and a healthy appetite for food). I really loved the changes in my body, especially when I started to feel my baby move. This didn't happen until I was about 15-16 weeks along. I'll never forget that moment.

Up to this point, I'd been paying careful attention to everything happening in my body. Other mama friends had told me that at first the feeling is like a flutter or gas bubbles. I had plenty of gas bubbles (one of the less glamorous aspects of pregnancy), but I knew this was different. The movement repeated several times and confirmed to me this was my baby. My heart swelled with pure joy. That was my baby! Moving inside me! After that I started feeling her move more and more.

I had so much fun watching my belly move around. It was a little creepy yet wonderful at the same time. The whole growing-another-human-inside-my-body concept has always seemed rather sci-fi to me.

During this trimester you'll notice the biggest changes in your body. Some might feel overwhelming, while others magical. Pay attention to each moment and enjoy the miracle manifesting within you.

MEDITATION & MINDFULNESS

Nothing will bring you into the present and into your body like childbirth. If you're not used to being aware of your body or focusing on the present moment, labor can be quite shocking. Learning how to practice mindfulness will come in handy for when the big day comes.

Mindfulness will also become an essential tool during those long nights and days post-baby when you feel like you'll never again have a moment to yourself. Learning to create quiet space for you will be a lifesaver. Raising a child can be an amazing tornado of magical chaos, but that doesn't mean you need to lose yourself in the madness.

For me practicing mindfulness was hard. My mind tends to dash into a thousand directions within a minute. Staying present was not an easy task. I began talking baby steps with focusing on my breath or counting my heartbeat for 60 counts. Sometimes, I just focused on chewing a bite of food. I paid attention to the flavors, texture, and the movement of my mouth.

Magical Goddess Tip:

Start small. Practice by counting to five while inhaling, hold for five, and exhale for five. Repeat 3 times and check with how you feel.

Sometimes though, I needed some more guidance. My favorite guided meditations are the 21-day Meditation Challenges by Deepak Chopra and Oprah. They are less than 20 minutes long, and fit perfect into a busy schedule. These meditations helped me heal from childbirth and rekindle my relationships after dealing with a bout of postpartum depression.

Journaling is also wonderful on its own, and as an excellent companion to meditation. Reflecting upon one's experience during this incredible period of transformation and change can create a keen sense of awareness. I now wished I'd written more in my pregnancy journal. Even if you only write one or two lines or mark a milestone, take the time to document the magic and capture those amazing moments.

Now is the time to establish a solid meditation practice and practice being present. There are so many resources out there for developing your mediation skills. Here are a few to get you started:
Chopra Meditation
www.chopximeditation.com
Gabriel Bernstein's book Miracles Now, Hayhouse
Yoga Journal
www.yogajournal.com/category/meditation/
GaiamTV
www.gaiamtv.com

LOVE YOUR BODY

Body image is a serious issue among women. Our society is inundated with ideas of what beauty is; what we should look like, what we should wear. Females have a tough time from the beginning as culture dictates what size we should be. Then we get pregnant and our body goes through some crazy changes as we grow a little human inside us.

I went from a size small to medium in the first six months of my pregnancy. I remember taking a shower and then trying to put on a pair of small underwear. I couldn't get them higher than mid-thigh. Not sure why I found this funny, but I nearly peed my pants laughing.

Oddly enough, I never felt more beautiful than when I was pregnant, despite my 50+ pound weight gain. I loved the way my body looked and would stare at my growing baby bump in the mirror every day, and for once in my life I had boobs! The new curves of my body made me feel sexy. I truly felt like a goddess: strong, beautiful, and radiant.

Sadly this is not every woman's experience. Often there is pressure to maintain a certain weight, regardless of the fact that pregnancy will result in some weight gain. "Bouncing back" after pregnancy has its own set of pressures too. That is why learning to love your body now is so important.

Think about how amazing your body is. During pregnancy, your body is actually creating, nourishing, and protecting the life (or lives) growing inside you. If you stop for a moment to contemplate the complexity of this phenomenon, it will blow your mind. Pregnancy is like an amazing sci-fi film taking place in real life. Inside you! At the same time, your body is keeping you healthy. You're likely to get less colds or illnesses during pregnancy, especially if you take good care of your body.

Building a healthy relationship with your body will motivate you to take better care of yourself during and after pregnancy. Once you do this, your body will reward you with a wonderful feeling of vibrancy which will perpetuate even more self-care. When you feel good, you feel better about yourself and how you look, and you will radiate beauty to the world.

Magical Goddess Tip:

Take a moment and look at yourself in the mirror. Look right into your eyes and say, "I am beautiful. I love you." Do this often, even if it feels silly at first. Say it until you believe it, because it's true.

You are beautiful and you are loved. You must love yourself in order to love those close to you. Loving yourself leads to proper self-care.

SELF-CARE

This is the time to establish great self-care habits that you can also use after the baby comes. Some mothers let themselves become so consumed with baby care they forget to take care of themselves. Some feel that putting their needs before those of the baby makes them selfish, or think that self-care is indulgent and wasteful, but true self-care is neither.

Self-care is taking care of your mind, body, and spirit so you can be the strong, balanced mother your family needs you to be. If you are feeling deprived, tired, stressed, or overwhelmed, it's time to take a close look at your life and determine the areas that are in need of attention. Ask yourself these questions and write an honest answer for each one in your journal:

- How many hours of sleep do I need? Am I getting those hours of rest every night or during a 24-hour period?
- Am I eating a balanced diet that includes whole grains, fresh fruits and vegetables, legumes and other quality protein sources? Am I eating too many sweets or junk food? What am I craving? What kind of nutrition is in the food I'm craving? (Note: Cravings usually signal a nutritional deficiency.)

- Am I stressed? Is it affecting my sleep? Is my job stressful? Am I taking five minutes to sit quietly and breathe every day? Do I go outside daily or spend a few minutes in nature?
- What am I feeling overwhelmed about? Is it the delivery or labor? Is it the home I live in? Are my friends and family stressing me out?
- What do I need right now? What makes me feel good? What calms me? What helps me get through a tough situation?

Look at your answers and develop a plan. Find what you have control over and can make changes necessary. Start a list of activities that can help you get to a better place mentally, physically, and spiritually. Make this list visible and easy for you to access later.

Here is an example of my top five self-care habits, which I had written on my bathroom mirror with a dry eraser pen for months until they became second nature:

1. Oil-pulling (swishing coconut oil in your mouth 15 minutes followed by a good brushing. WebMD has a great article: http://www.webmd.com/oral-health/features/oil-pulling)
2. Go outside
3. Dance to a song
4. 15 minutes of yoga
5. 5-10 minutes of meditation

I try to do everything on that list every day. Sometimes I combine yoga and time outside by going out on our spacious balcony with my daughter to do yoga while she plays. Often times she joins me in the yoga. She especially loves downward facing dog pose. She also loves to dance with me to electronic dance music, which is beyond adorable.

Going through several bouts of postpartum depression, I learned quickly the importance of self-care. When I'm stressed out, I like to take a bath with my favorite essential oils and sea salts. A fifteen minute bath helps I feel relaxed, refreshed, and recharged. If I'm craving junk food, I consider what maybe is missing from my diet and make sure I eat foods as rich in that nutrient as possible. For example, if I'm craving sugar, I'll eat a bowl of pasta with freshly chopped veggies and shredded cheese. This combination of foods works well to give me the proper nourishment to boost my energy level. Speaking of veggies, I'm not a huge fan. Sounds strange coming from a vegetarian, but I'll only eat a huge bowl of salad if I have a yummy dressing and some fresh bread to go with it, or a veggie platter if there is a tasty ranch dip available.

If I feel frumpy, I take a look in the mirror and ask myself why. Sometimes all I need is a shower, a quick hair brushing, or on a little makeup. Other times I feel the need for more drastic intervention, such as getting a massage, pedicure, or facial. If our budget is tight, I give myself a lymphatic massage (see the end of section), put a moisturizing/cleansing mask on my face made from ingredients I have on hand, or paint my toenails (although in the later stages of pregnancy this maybe difficult).

Here are some quick beauty treatments you can do at home:

Egg White Mask

Remove the yolk from an uncooked egg and apply the remaining whites to your face with a cosmetic brush. Let dry (5-10 minutes). Wash face. Enjoy smooth, firm skin. Do this routine 2-3 days in a row to clear acne.

Cucumber Mask

Take the peels from a cucumber and rub them across your face. Cucumbers help hydrate and tone the skin. You can also blend a cucumber, add a few drops of fresh lemon juice, and apply to face to help lighten skin. Rinse after 5 minutes.

Oatmeal Mask

Blend dry oatmeal into a coarse powder. Mix with water until you achieve paste-like consistency. Apply to face and let dry. Use a wet washcloth to remove mask. Oatmeal is a great base for exfoliation.

Sugar Body Scrub

Mix 1 cup of brown sugar in ½-1 cup of jojoba oil. Apply generously to body, especially dry areas like knees and elbows while in shower. Rinse (you may need a little soap if your skin feels too oily). Enjoy soft, moisturized skin.

Lymphatic Body Massage

Brush, as if dusting off dirt, every area of your body three times starting with the opposite arm. Lightly brush your fingertips from your hand toward the elbow on both sides (inner and outer arm). Continue upward from your elbow to shoulder. When both arms are done, brush the inside of your armpits downward. Now brush the back of your neck, moving from the top of your head to the nape of neck. Continue toward your face. Using both hands on either side, start from the center of the forehead, brushing around the eyes, down the cheeks to the jaw, and moving back to the top of your nose. Brush at the inside of the eyes down around your mouth ending at the tip of the chin. Brush your neck to the collarbone and across the chest. Brush the sides of your neck to the end of the shoulders.

Make the figure eight sign around your breasts and brush down the sides of your body to the hips. Make circles over your belly starting from the right side moving towards the left. Brush either side of your lower back down to the buttocks. Make circles on either glut moving inward toward the sacrum.

Move to the back of the knees and brush upwards toward the gluts. Do the same to the sides of your thighs and the front of the knees and lower legs. Avoid the interior legs during pregnancy due to higher risk of blood clots. Continue the same with the lower legs starting from the ankles moving to the knees and then the tops of the toes to the ankles.

Take a deep breath and a moment to notice how great your body feels now. This simple massage practice can be done in five minutes and is so effective in releasing stress. Moving the lymph in your body stimulates your immune system. The lymphatic system doesn't have a pumping mechanism as the circulatory (the heart) does, therefore moving the lymph is important to maintain your health. Physical exercise also helps with the circulation of the lymph. This massage gives you an opportunity to show your body some much needed love and can benefit post-birth moms with water retention.

Magical Goddess Tip:

Do at least one thing every day that makes you feel like a goddess.

CHILDBIRTH CLASSES

There are many classes to choose from when it comes to child-birth. If you are planning a hospital birth, they will recommend their classes. Birthing centers also offer a variety of classes, mostly focusing on natural child-birth and breathing techniques.

I made the grave mistake of thinking, "I'm a woman. I have intuition. I've witnessed live births (both in hospital and home), and I'll know what I need to do." and chose to forego the traditional birthing classes. I took the *Birthing From Within* class based on the book by Pam England from the birthing center, which were interesting. We practiced several exercises holding ice and using different breathing/meditation techniques to endure the pain. I did okay and thought, "See, I can deal with pain. I totally have this under control."

The closer I got to the delivery, the more ill-prepared I felt. While this is a common emotion for expectant mamas, even those who've had previous pregnancies, I knew I should have taken more informational classes. But we were getting close to the end of my pregnancy and out of time. I went into labor two weeks before my due date and ended up missing half of the classes I had signed up for, including a breast-feeding class I had really wanted to take.

It's important to register for and take classes towards the end of the second trimester beginning of the third. I waited too long and missed out on a lot of helpful information that would have eased my transition into motherhood. Knowledge is power, in my opinion. You'll need to find a balance in scheduling the classes, because you don't want to do them too soon and then forget the valuable information before you have the baby.

You can read everything on natural childbearing, watch every birthing film out there, and attend every single class your community has to offer, but when the labor pains kick in, much of what you've learned goes out the window. That's where doulas play an important role at the time labor and delivery. I'll talk more about that in the section entitled Doula.

Right now, find some classes that interest you, signup, and take them. Here are some sites with more information about various classes:

Birthing From Within
http://www.birthingfromwithin.com/

HypnoBirthing
http://www.hypnobirthing.com/

Bradley Birth
http://www.bradleybirth.com/

MATERNITY CLOTHES

You might have noticed that your clothes no longer fit you as well as they did a month or two ago. By 10 weeks I couldn't wear any of my pants. I needed a new wardrobe, especially professional clothes for work.

Lucky for me, a dear friend offered to take me shopping as she knew some great consignment shops in our area. She helped me pick out clothes that worked for my tight budget. Unfortunately for me, there were few items in my size at the consignment stores so we ended up at Motherhood Maternity outlet store.

I had a $300 budget to spend on clothes, and I needed both professional and casual outfits. Here is what I bought:

2 pairs of black slacks
2 pairs of jeans
1 pair of yoga pants
1 pair of workout capris
1 pair of black capris
4 solid colored short-sleeved shirts
1 black dress
2 fun tops

The solid-colored tops could be mixed and matched with black slacks for work. I threw a cardigan or a light shrug over them to make it look more professional. A couple of my mama friends also gave me some of their clothes. Between what I purchased and what was given to me, I had a simple wardrobe that I love and met my needs. As I lost my pregnancy weight in the months after my daughter was born, I was actually sad to pack away my maternity clothes. I enjoyed having a limited set of outfits and the extra space in my closet.

A few tips when shopping for maternity clothes:

If you are a size medium in your pre-pregnancy clothes, then you buy size medium maternity wear. However, toward the end of your pregnancy, you may need to move up a size.

Make sure whatever you buy is comfortable. Things will get tighter as you get bigger, and, potentially, more uncomfortable.

Plan for the seasons. If you are due in winter, make sure you purchase maternity clothes that can be layered for comfort. My daughter was due in January, but I stayed with a warm weather wardrobe because my pregnancy hormones had me cooking like an oven. If I did get cold, I just tossed a cardigan over what I already had on and left it unbuttoned.

Bellybands. I discovered this awesome invention of clothing through a friend when she sent me a few of hers. They are elastic cloth bands that are worn over regular pants to extend the life of your non-maternity wardrobe. You can leave the pants unbuttoned and place the band over the top part to keep them from falling down as you move throughout your day. When worn with a maternity top, it simply looks like you have a layered shirt underneath. They come in many of colors and fabrics. You can find them on eBay, Amazon, and Motherhood Maternity.

Shoes. Make sure you have a solid pair of shoes that provide decent arch support. Toward the end of your pregnancy your feet may swell. When that time comes, a pair of comfortable sandals or quality flip-flops will come in handy.

There are so many stylish maternity clothes now, it's easy to get carried away. Start with the basics listed above.

Magical Goddess Tip:

Don't be afraid to treat yourself to that cute outfit that makes you feel gorgeous, but is a bit pricey. Remember you will never be pregnant with this baby(s) again. Give yourself permission to splurge a little.

PREPARING YOUR HOME

Bringing a new life into your home can create havoc. One of the first things I told my husband after the positive pregnancy test was that I wanted our carpet torn out and hardwood floors put in. We'd wanted to do this since we first moved into our condo, but replacing the flooring while living there was no easy feat, so we kept putting the project off. However, when we discovered our little munchkin would be joining the household, we could no longer delay the project.

The carpet was brand-new when we moved in, but with two cats, I didn't want our child crawling on the same floor where the cats often puked. We waited until I had gotten over the morning sickness, because I knew I couldn't tolerate any more stress during that time. It took about three months but we finally did it. Two years later, I still love the IKEA floors we put in. Wiping up vomit from the cats or the baby is a breeze, and keeping them clean is so easy compared to the carpeting.

Changing our floors is just one example that we took to make our home more practical for the baby. Each home is different and each family has their own preference. Think about what you need to create a comfortable, nurturing space for you and your baby.

Preparing your home also means making room for baby. Now is a great time to de-clutter those closets and get rid of the stuff in your home that you don't use or enjoy. We got rid of our futon and replaced it with two rocking leather recliners. A comfortable place to sit was a true blessing during long nights of teething or fevers.

Magical Goddess Tip:

Start small when decluttering and make it a daily ritual. For example, take 5-10 minutes each day to clear out a small area such as a cupboard, counter, or drawer. If you have a lot of stuff to sort through, taking smaller steps will make the process less daunting.

We also invested in some quality storage cabinets to organize our stuff since our condo lacked adequate storage to accommodate an additional person's belongings. We made room for the baby while creatively managing the space available.

Preparing the kitchen is central to a smooth postpartum period. We invested in a Vitamix blender which I used frequently while going through postpartum depression, since I had zero appetite, my husband was able to make high-calorie smoothies to ensure I got the nutrients needed to maintain my milk supply. The blender also came in handy for baby food later on.

We also purchased in a high-quality glass storage container set to portion our food and store homemade baby food. They were also great for storing leftovers because they are safe for freezing and reheating. I love to can so I made my favorite jellies, sauces, and pickles. My husband canned a whole bunch of applesauce which came in handy the following year when our girl started eating solids.

Baby-Proofing. Start looking at your house to see what needs to be done to ensure a safe environment for your little one. You can baby-proof very inch of your home and still not achieve a 100 % kid-safe zone. There also parents who think that their child should learn to live in a normal environment from the beginning. Whichever mindset you find yourself in, here are two things you can do that are easy and will make a difference: wall socket plugs and cabinet locks. Eventually your child will figure them out, but they will provide some measure of peace of mind.

Check out IKEA and The Container Store for some great organizing and space-saving tips. Here's a great article on nursery organization from Apartment Therapy: http://www.apartmenttherapy.com/nursery-organization-tips-from-apartment-therapy-readersnesting-a-nursery-168614

PART THREE

Third Trimester

Congratulations, mama! You've made it to the last leg of this amazing, magical journey. I want you to take a moment and check in with your body and your little baby. Place your left hand over your heart center and your right hand over your belly. Allow the energy of love in your heart to travel through your left hand up your arm, across your shoulders, down your right arm, into your right hand, and out over your belly. Surround your baby with light. Allow this cocoon of love to encompass you as well. Treasure this moment connecting with your baby. In a few short months you'll be meeting your little angel.

When you are ready turn your focus on your body. How are you feeling? Check in with each area of your body. Are there any areas of discomfort? Take a deep breath and release the tension you might find. When you are finished take a moment to jot down this experience in your journal.

You might be feeling very pregnant now. Or you might be one of the few people who have gorgeous slender waists that tend to hide the baby somewhere like a TARDIS or Hermione's purse. One such example is a neighbor I had growing up. When she went into labor with her fourth child, the hospital nurse wanted to transfer her to the high-risk maternity ward because she "couldn't possibly be nine months pregnant." My friend almost delivered her kid right there at the nurse's station. She had gone from a size 4 to a size 6 at the end of her pregnancy, never ever wore maternity clothes. If you are not one of these types of people, do not worry. I know I felt like a beached whale when I hit my 8th month.

As you enter the last trimester it may be hard to believe you have come this far, but here you are, finishing up the last few projects, getting the nursery together, and preparing for the big show. Perhaps you've had a baby shower, your relatives and friends are getting antsy to meet your little angel, and you are starting to feel the reality of your pregnancy even more now.

During the last two months of pregnancy I started feeling very uncomfortable. My pelvis hurt and I had to visit a prenatal chiropractor every week to get adjusted. Yes, there are chiropractors who specialize in prenatal care, and they are miracle workers! I'd hobble in, feeling like my pelvis was about to split in two, and walk out fifteen minutes later feeling like I could run a marathon.

My feet started swelling too, so every night after I came home, I had to put them up. My midwife had me drinking coconut water every day and that seemed to help.

My husband and I took a few last weekend trips up to Seattle, and also went to the beach because we knew we wouldn't be able to do so for a while.

Sleep became a thing of the past. I started waking up in the middle of the night, not just to pee, but also from insomnia. My midwife said this was natural, that my body was preparing me for the crazy baby schedule I'd be on for the next couple of years. Nearly a year after my daughter was born, I read an article stating that researchers have found that many mothers start exhibiting postpartum depression symptoms well before the baby is born. Insomnia is one of those signs. People kept telling me I needed to sleep as much as possible. Because I worked 10-hour days, I didn't have time to nap except for a 30-minute rest at lunch time. After a couple of emotional meltdowns due to exhaustion, I started to go to bed right after I ate dinner. I didn't care if I woke up in the middle of the night, because I would wake up regardless, so I got sleep when I could. The early bedtime helped tremendously.

I also experienced "pregnancy brain syndrome." Yes, it's real and if you haven't experienced it yet, it's possible you will after the baby arrives. My writing took a big hit due to pregnancy brain. I used to be able to crank out 3,000-5,000 words in one sitting after working all day, but shortly after I got pregnant, writing 500 words felt like I'd done a marathon swim across the Pacific during a typhoon. My memory was shot and I couldn't remember anything. Postpartum depression only made it worse. It took two years to get back into writing fiction again.

As you near the end of this magical journey, you'll notice many changes in yourself and your body. This is the time to get last minute things done, because it won't be long before you're holding your sweet bundle in your arms, mama. You'll need all the support you can get.

DOULA

A doula is a professional birth coach who will support the mother emotionally and physically. She can also guide the mother's partner in supporting her as well. They are not medical professionals and do not assist with the actual birth, but are there throughout to help the mother with her breathing and laboring positions. Research has shown that women with a doula present at their labor and delivery tend to have less medical interventions, like medication for pain relief and C-sections. (Hodnett ED, Gates S, Hofmeyr GJ, Sakala C. Continuous Support for Women During Childbirth. Cochrane Database of Systematic Reviews. (3) CD003766, 2003.)

This is one thing I regret not doing. I had several friends who were doulas and offered to help, but I declined figuring that between my midwife and her two assistants, I had plenty of support. It was after I'd had a vacuum-assisted delivery, in the hospital, with an epidural, that I realized my mistake.

When my husband told me his side of the experience, I realized that he had no idea what he should be doing. The doula's job is to help the mom but also to coach the dad or partner how to better support the mom. He said he felt so helpless, and that the whole thing felt like a nightmare. He told me that the entire time we were at the birthing center, he felt lost. He desperately wanted to help me but didn't know how so he left the room feeling completely helpless. I remember when he did this and how lonely I felt without him there. A doula would have given him a job to do.

Back in the day, midwives came to deliver babies at home and all the women of the family would gather around to hold up the laboring mother. They were the doulas giving the mother the emotional support she needed to birth a child. Today we don't have that village approach to birth; we have doulas.

I know if I ever choose to have another child, I will definitely hire a doula. They can be expensive, but you can always hire a newly-graduated doula who charges on donation basis. As a new grad, they need to attend a certain number of births to obtain certification.

For more information check out the following links:

American Pregnancy Organization

http://americanpregnancy.org/labor-and-birth/having-a-doula/

DONA

http://www.dona.org/mothers/

FINDING A PEDIATRICIAN

Now is the time to start looking for a good pediatrician. I didn't do any research beforehand and things got a little crazy once our baby arrived. The one I settled on is adequate. She knows her stuff and allows me to make the necessary choices for my child without being too pushy. She wasn't a mother herself when we first met, but now she is and our relationship has changed for the better. Like finding the right provider for your prenatal care, it is equally important to find a pediatrician that matches your values and lifestyle but also you and your child feel comfortable.

Word of mouth is a great way to find an excellent provider, so ask around. I found my pediatrician through a reference from one of the nurses who took care of me in the postnatal unit at the hospital. There was a clinic had I wanted to take my daughter to because I knew several families I knew took their kids there, and had always raved about how wonderful they were, but the clinic was too far from our home. Consider the ease and accessibility of the clinic you choose.

Write a list of what is important to you and start researching. Many clinics have their physicians' profiles up on their website. Here are a few things to think about:

- Staff coverage and hours
- Vaccination schedule (some clinics may have strict policies regarding vaccination)
- Openness to holistic health
- How emergencies are handled
- After-hours availability
- Access to health info and physicians/nurses online

Make sure you have more than one provider in mind, because sometimes the first one doesn't work out. After two years under our current pediatrician care, we're moving to a different provider in the same practice, not because we don't like her, but it turns out my daughter is terrified of women physicians and does better with male doctors. You want to make sure you find someone you can trust with the care of your child.

PREPARING YOURSELF

There are many ways to prepare yourself before the baby's arrival, one of which is to take time for yourself. Once the baby arrives, your days will be so full that finding time for yourself can be difficult. Focus on self-care but on a bigger scale. Treat yourself to a massage or pedicure. Get your hair done. Buy yourself that piece of jewelry you've been eyeing for months. Do something nice for yourself.

Go to the movies. Enjoy date nights with your spouse or partner. Have lunch with your girlfriends. Read the book you've wanted to read. Enjoy your life and do whatever brings you joy or makes you feel good.

For me, that meant getting my legs professionally waxed so I didn't have to worry about shaving before labor began. The last couple of weeks, I took it easy. Besides a yoga video or swimming at the gym, I relaxed at home and leisurely organized all the newborn clothes I'd received. The best gift my husband gave me that year was monthly series of prenatal massages. I went to two different therapists that I loved. Each one added her own magical touch of healing for my body.

Focus on your home too. Make sure you have meals available for you and your family for the first couple of weeks to a month after the baby comes. People may be willing to bring food, so find someone trustworthy to set up a meal train. Fill your freezer with yummy, quick, microwavable meals, and your refrigerator with easy snacks you can eat with one hand, since you'll be holding a newborn with the other.

Ideas for snacks: cheese sticks, hummus, veggie sticks, yogurt, yogurt smoothies, kefir, fruits, crackers, protein bars, premade smoothies, sandwich fixings, etc.

Go through all of the baby things people have given you or you've gotten from the shower and get them organized. I organized all of my daughter's clothes by size and put them in labeled bins. A friend suggested programming a reminder on my phone calendar every three months to rotate the clothes out because you may forget otherwise.

Download a good baby care app to your phone that will help you keep track of the baby's feeding/peeing/pooping schedule. They'll want you to do this at the hospital to make sure the baby is getting enough to eat. Also download a good white noise app. This will come in handy during baby nap time.

Magical Goddess Tip:

Create a volunteer schedule for the first few weeks for people who offer to help with things like running errands, housekeeping, laundry or watching the baby while you nap.

Here are a couple of blog posts I did about pre-baby prep:
10 Things You Should Do When You Are Pregnant
http://www.melaniatolan.com/2013/11/10-things-you-should-do-when-you-are.html

Smartphone Apps for New Moms
http://www.melaniatolan.com/2015/05/smartphone-apps-for-new-moms.html

BIRTH PLAN

"Why the hell would I need a birth plan?" I muttered to myself when I read about them in a pregnancy article online. My "birth plan" was to have my baby at the birthing center and then go home the next day; a natural water birth attended by my midwife and her two lovely assistants. My husband would be there to massage my back and hold my hand during contractions. I didn't need anyone else.

After actually giving birth, in a way that was completely different than what I'd imagined, I contemplated how the hell I'd ended up here. Not that I was sad to be in the hospital, on the contrary, for me the hospital had been a blessing. What I questioned was the feeling of being lost that filled every crevice of my body and mind. I didn't know what to do next because I hadn't planned for this at all.

Having a birth plan didn't seem like such a bad idea now. How I wished I'd written one, even for the midwives, to let them know what I needed and hoped for. I learned that it never hurts to have a plan, no matter where or what type of birth you are planning, just make sure that being flexible is an integral part of that plan.

Think about what you want and figure out what your options are. Talk to your provider and ask questions regarding their approach to a birth plan. Discuss with your partner what you are willing and not willing to do in various scenarios and then write in down.

Magical Goddess Tip:

Give a copy to your provider, your doula (if you are using one), your emergency contact person, and tuck one copy in your hospital/birth bag.

Here are some websites that have great information and sample birth plans:
Earth Mama Angel Baby
http://www.earthmamaangelbaby.com/free-birth-plan
Mama Natural
http://www.mamanatural.com/wp-content/uploads/2010/06/MamaNatural_Birth_Plan.pdf
Baby Center
http://assets.babycenter.com/ims/Content/my_birth_plan.pdf

BREASTFEEDING

Your breasts have probably increased in size by now. I remember looking down at my chest and gasping, "I have boobs!" For the first time in my life, I was busting out of my bra. I wanted to jump for joy. I loved looking at myself in the mirror and pointing out to my dear husband that his wife finally had some nice ta-tas. He smiled and said, "If I'd known you'd be this sexy pregnant, I'd have knocked you up a long time ago."

As much as I loved my new boobs, I knew the reason why they'd doubled in size and I looked forward to putting them to work. I'm not going to go into all the details of why breastfeeding is best, or try to convince you to breastfeed if you are thinking otherwise. There are enough websites, articles, books, and other informational sources that will tell you everything you need to know to make the decision that is best for you.

If you are planning on breastfeeding, now is the time to take a class or two offered by either the hospital or the birthing center near you. I waited way too long to sign up for my class, and I actually went into labor the day I was supposed to attend. I thought, "Gosh, I'll just trust my intuition and I'll know what to do."

Well, it turns out I didn't know what to do, and I struggled for many weeks after I delivered. Thankfully I had wonderful lactation specialists in the hospital that helped me out during the first few days who were also available by phone and email after I went home. Having some knowledge prior to the birth would have helped. I encourage you to find a class and read up on breastfeeding basics because once the baby is here you won't have the luxury of time.

If you are planning to return to work while breastfeeding, you will need a pump. A friend gave me her 10-year-old Medela pump, and it worked fine for me. Pumps are expensive, but you can find used ones on Craigslist or eBay. Don't forget to check with your insurance because sometimes they will reimburse you for part or the full price you paid for a new pump.

Nursing bras or tanks are good to have on hand, however keep in mind your breasts will increase in size once your milk comes in. I bought a bra that adjusted in size and a nursing tank, which worked perfectly for me, but for women larger than a C cup, you might want to look for a bra that gives you the necessary support.

Visit Nordstrom's or Motherhood Maternity to try out different bras. You don't have to purchase them there. Often times you can find them at Nordstrom Rack or online liquidation sites like www.zulily.com. What you want to look for is comfort and support. Beware of underwire or constraining bras as they can lead to mastitis (clogged ducts) later when you are producing milk.

Night nursing bras are important because you want to be comfortable and have easy access. I know bras with snaps were too much fuss for me at night so the overlapping bras worked best for me.

You may also need nursing pads. I thought I would be the Zen mama who only uses organic cotton reusable nursing pads. I even had some on my baby registry and someone actually bought them for me. However, I discovered they didn't work so well for me at the beginning because they stuck to the raw spots on my nipples. I soon switched over to disposables when I developed thrush from the antibiotics I received at the hospital and had to change pads after every feeding. I used the disposables for several months, however, when my daughter was about 14 months, started using the organic cotton ones again. I liked them because I only needed one at night and then I could wash them with my girl's laundry every couple of days or so.

For more information about breastfeeding education and products, check out these websites:

Kelly Mom
http://kellymom.com/
La Leche League

http://www.llli.org/
The documentary: *Breastmilk* www.breastmilkthemovie.com

HOSPITAL/BIRTH BAG

Whether you are planning to deliver at home, the hospital or a birthing center, you should pack a birth bag. Why? Because having the essential items you need during labor and delivery at your fingertips will reduce a lot of chaos and stress. Also if there is a chance you need to go to the hospital for any reason, you're already packed and ready to go. Anytime after 30 weeks is a good time to start thinking about what you'll need.

Here's what to pack:

For you:
- Toiletries (toothbrush, toothpaste, deodorant, your favorite body wash and shampoo, and lotion),
- Hair brush or comb
- Ties for long hair
- Lip balm
- 2 changes of your most comfy lounge-wear like yoga pants and a soft top or a sweat set
- Comfortable pajamas that are breastfeeding-friendly
- Nursing pads and nipple cream

- 2 pairs of underwear (the hospital will most likely give you a pair, but in case you want to wear your own, best to have them available)
- 2 nursing bras (night nursing bras or tanks are fine and likely the most comfortable to wear at this time)
- A robe
- Slippers and flip-flops
- A going home outfit for mama
- Phone charger
- Your favorite relaxing music, or meditation CD or MP3 player

For Baby:
- A going home outfit for baby
- Newborn diapers and wipes (the hospital will most likely provide these to you, but it never hurts to throw in a few for the ride home)
- Newborn hat
- Baby blanket
- A couple of receiving blankets

Misc:
- Healthy snacks for your partner and you later on. The hospital and birthing centers will feed you but sometimes you need to munch on something in the middle of the night or after a nursing session
- Change of clothes for your partner
- Toiletries for partner

For more ideas on what to pack for the hospital check out this website:

Pregnant Chicken

http://www.pregnantchicken.com/pregnant-chicken-blog/2012/5/21/hospital-bag-what-to-pack.html

POSTPARTUM DEPRESSION

This is something that isn't talked about nearly enough during the prenatal period, and I believe that it is vitally important to discuss, especially now. During my pregnancy, my midwives only mentioned depression a couple of times in passing, and I wish they'd given me more information during my prenatal visits so I could have read up on the condition.

Many women experience emotional lows right after birth as the body readjusts its hormone levels. This is often referred to as "baby blues" and can last a couple of weeks, sometimes longer.

During this time, a new mama can feel sad, cry for no reason, be unable to sleep, and/or have a loss of appetite. Mild symptoms are considered normal, and good self-care can help tremendously. However, if these symptoms continue, and/or become more severe, please consult your provider immediately.

I didn't know that I was becoming depressed and dismissed the signs as me being a "weak mom." Yes, motherhood can be difficult, but it shouldn't be a constant struggle. Reach out and get the help you need. You are not weak for doing so, nor are you a failure for needing assistance. Remember, it takes a village to raise a child, so find your village and your mama tribe.

Now is a good time to join or make contacts in a mama's group, preferably with mamas that are due in the same season as you. These relationships will come in handy and nourish you later on after baby arrives. This will be your mama tribe and now is the time to cultivate these vital relationships.
- Know the signs of postpartum depression:
- Mood swings
- Constant sadness
- Irritability and intense anger
- Excessive crying
- Lack of concentration
- Loss of appetite
- Insomnia
- Fatigue
- Difficulty bonding with your baby
- Withdrawal from others

Dark thoughts including harming yourself or the baby

Look into hiring a postpartum doula, someone who can come and care for you and your baby, preferably at night so you can get the needed rest. The DONA website has a directory of doulas in your area.

Magical Goddess Tip:

Learn to be gentle with yourself. There will be many sleepless nights. Don't judge yourself for not doing what you think you "should" be doing or assume that you are doing things wrong.

All mamas do what they can with the resources they have available. When things get rough, remember this phase will pass. Things will get better.

Here are some books to read on PPD:

Down Came the Rain by Brooke Shields, Hyperion.

The Mommy Myth: The Idealization of Motherhood and How It Has Undermined Women by Susan J. Douglas and Meredith Michaels, Simon and Schuster.

Also check out these websites:

Postpartum Progress

http://www.postpartumprogress.com/

Postpartum Support International

www.pospartum.net

THE BLESSING WAY

As I mentioned in the birthing class section, I read *Birthing from Within* by Pam England, and it was the first time I heard of a "blessing way ceremony." The moment I read about it, I knew I had to have one. Luckily my Wise Sisters were already planning one for me. This simple ceremony and gathering of women was one of the most magical moments in my pregnancy.

A blessing way is a party for the mama-to-be where she gets pampered and experiences a few rituals. It's kind of like a shower for the mommy celebrating her transition into mommyhood.

At mine, the women saged me, drew beautiful designs on my belly with henna, gave me a lovely Reiki session, and made a beaded bracelet for me to wear until after I gave birth. They brought my favorite foods, desserts, and chocolate. For an entire two hours, I felt like a goddess queen. All the women present were mothers and each of them contributed a bead for my bracelet. Having that bracelet with me during the early stages of my labor brought much comfort.

Here are some ideas for a blessing way ceremony:

Invite only the women you are 100 percent comfortable with, like your best friends or extended family members. Include someone you look up to, such as friend who is a mother already. You want to have only positive mommy energy around you at this time. Appoint this person to be the leader or organizer.

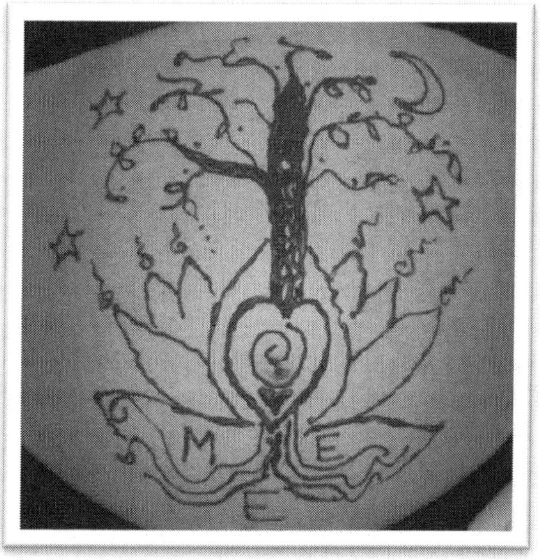

Figure 1 My beautiful henna belly.

Rituals. Talk to your lead person about what you want as far as rituals. You can do whatever you want but let the women surprise you with a ritual as well. Examples of some rituals are: saging, henna belly art, belly casting, jewelry making, Reiki or energy work, foot bath, creating a labyrinth, body painting, web-weaving, or creating a piece of art to commemorate the ceremony.

Candles. At my friend's blessing way, we each got votive candles that we lit at our own homes on the day she had her C-section.

Food. As I mentioned about my blessing way, the ladies brought my favorite foods.

Gifts. It is up to you whether you want to receive gifts but know that people love to give. Perhaps make the theme something like "A Day at the Spa" and each person can bring a spa product or "Nail Polish Fest" and someone can give you a mini pedicure as part of the ritual.

Magical Goddess Tip:

Allow yourself to receive the love. This event is about you, mama.

There are so many ways to make this ceremony fun and enjoyable, but most of all magical.

Mystic Mama
http://www.mysticmamma.com/blessing-way/
Blessing Way Book
http://www.blessingwaybook.com/

EPILOGUE

I hope this book has provided some valuable basic information to help you on your magical journey into motherhood. This is a beautiful time of change and transformation, but sometimes things don't always go as planned. Just when you think you've got everything figured out or under control, a bump in the road may occur. If that happens, know that it's all part of the journey. We are never 100% in control because this is another human being growing inside of us. They have feeling, opinions, and ideas too. They are as much of an individual as you are.

Our job as mothers is to hold space for that little creature to come into their own. There will be ups and there will be downs, but that's how it goes. There is perfection in imperfection. Mamas always question themselves and second-guess their decisions. This is normal and it doesn't make you a bad mother. Or less of a goddess. You, my dear, are an amazing woman.

Many blessings to you, mother goddess, and to your beautiful child too.

ACKNOWLEDGEMENTS

Thank you to my Sister Circle. You inspire me to follow my dreams and have always had my back. A thousand thank yous to each one of you.

Nicole, you are one kickass editor. Thank you for helping me hone my writing skills. Love you girl!

Maria, you have been with me from the beginning of my publishing journey. Thank you for all the editorial support.

Nadine and Susan, my first beta-readers, you gave me the courage to continue this project when it was barebones. Your feedback was worth the gold in Fort Knox.

And another thank you, Susan, for modeling your beautiful pregnant belly. You were the embodiment of a radiant urban goddess mama-to-be. Congrats on your little angel.

Christy, you are my cover fairy godmother. Thank you for creating yet another breathtaking cover.

My dear mother, you provided me with recipes for this book and teaching me how to use natural ingredients for beauty. You are my mama goddess. Thank you also for taking care of Boo Creature so I could work on this book. I love you and dad so much.

The biggest thank you goes to my man, Eric, who has been my rock and #1 fan. Thank you for giving me the gift of Boo and holding me when I'm falling apart. Thank you for believing in me. I love you, sweetheart.

ABOUT THE AUTHOR

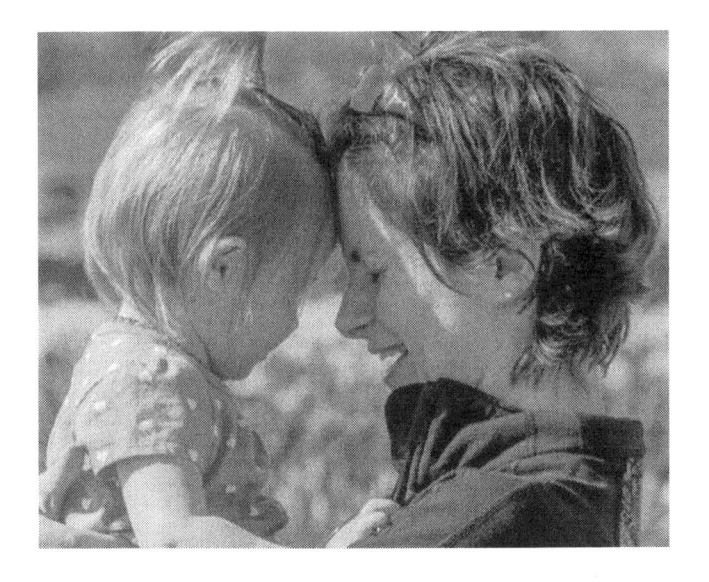

Melania can be found wearing comfy yoga pants in her modest kitchen stirring a boiling pot of organic pasta, feeding little Boo Creature fresh veggies, balancing a phone between her shoulder and cheek, all the while petting one of her feline beasts with a foot. She has been known to dance an Irish jig. You can also find her at www.melaniatolan.com.

Author of *Urban Goddess Mama- How I Got My Goddess Back After Postpartum Depression.*
Available here.

Enjoy the 1st chapter of **Urban *Goddess* Mama**- How I Got My Goddess Back After Postpartum Depression

By *Melania Tolan*

CHAPTER ONE

New Beginnings

Let me start from the beginning and give you a little background on my life. At age 33, I had everything going my way. I had a new career with the opportunity to work from home, a budding writing career by night, a fabulous husband who loved me exactly the way I was, and a cozy home in the city of Portland. I was surrounded by fantastic family and friends. All of these things made me feel like maybe I was ready to start a family.

I'd always been healthy. I exercised, kept a relaxed vegetarian diet, and made sure I got my eight hours of sleep every night. My spiritual life was thriving as I had joined a wonderful group of women years before who inspired me to add magic and beauty every single day. I meditated and prayed. Yoga was my best friend. I spent time outdoors, something not hard to do in the beautiful Pacific Northwest.

So when I decided to get pregnant, I envisioned myself as the all-natural, crunchy-granola, earth mama: bathed in glowing light, wearing flowing natural fiber clothing, my infant close to my breast in a Moby wrap as I strolled through the farmers' market filling my fair-trade basket with organic vegetables and herbs. Grace would become my middle name, and everyone I encountered would be blessed by my radiance. Oh yes! I was full of delusions of grandeur.

But that is where the fairytale ends and the true story begins. It was the Friday before Memorial Day 2012.

All week I'd been eating like a proper little piggy. One day I actually went to the cafeteria at work five times and bought full meals. This was in addition to filling my plate at the department potluck because I was so hungry. One of my coworkers teased, "You're pregnant. Ha ha."

Ha ha indeed.

That Friday I woke up at three a.m., my coworker's words echoing in my ears. Oh boy, what if she was right? I remembered I had a pregnancy test stuffed under the bathroom sink and practically jumped out of bed with anticipation. For the first time in my life of peeing on the "stick," it came out positive. I sucked in my breath as the plus sign filled the tiny window. *Here we go.*

I'd always known that when the time came to have a baby, I'd want a natural birth (obviously) either at home or at a birthing center. I'd watched *The Business of Being Born* and knew I was a healthy person who wouldn't need to be in the hospital.

When I found out I was pregnant, it seemed natural for me to pick a midwife and birthing center. I went with a local midwifery center, which came highly recommended by a personal friend and other acquaintances. Over the nine months of pregnancy, I received top-notch care from the nurse practitioner midwife and her two assistants. My only hang-up was that none of these women had children, but I squashed that feeling and didn't say anything because I liked them very much.

I was happy and reassured when my ultrasounds and labs throughout the pregnancy were normal. This validated the decision to have my baby at the birthing center rather than the hospital.

I had one appointment at the beginning of my pregnancy with the obstetrics office I used just to make sure everything would be okay. They also did all my ultrasounds. Originally I was supposed to see Dr. B, but the appointment had to be rescheduled because of an emergency procedure she was called away to perform.

I was bummed because I really liked her. She treated her patients well, and, being a mother herself, she understood what they went through. Instead I saw her partner, Dr. D. He'd delivered many of my friends' babies and operated on some of them, too. I trusted him and his opinion, and he reassured me everything looked fine with me and Baby.

Later that year in December, my husband and I took a *Birthing From Within* childbirth class, and we really enjoyed it. I discovered I could cope with pain well, as we had to hold ice in our hands while practicing the breathing techniques taught in class. I even bought the book that the class was based on and found it insightful. The art exercises were particularly helpful in dealing with the anxiety leading up to the actually birth. Yet I couldn't quite shrug the feeling something was missing or that I didn't feel very prepared. I kept telling myself these emotions were normal for new moms.

In my head, I had this vision of myself laboring in a luxurious tub filled with warm water at the birth center while my midwife coached me through the birth. I'd swum throughout most of the pregnancy and even wrote a mermaid young-adult novel over the summer so it only seemed appropriate that my daughter would be born in the water. Yeah, I was going to be the ultimate Zen water goddess mama, surrounded by candlelight and tranquility as I brought my little princess into the world.

The last trimester flew by like a torpedo, as we were busy with the holidays and getting everything ready for Baby to come the first week in February. My pelvis had been hurting badly, and I'd been going to see the chiropractor regularly for adjustment. However, the treatment on Friday, January 18, didn't seem to do much good, which worried me a bit.

My midwife was gone for a long weekend, but I wasn't concerned because this was my first baby and firstborns always come late. The next day, Saturday, I had my last prenatal massage. On Sunday, Hubby and I attended an infant CPR and first aid class.

Before the class, I went for a nice, relaxing swim. I swam longer than usual, and felt great. On the way home, I stopped by the store and bought some last minute items—just in case. That night, I finished up a book review for my blog, completed some other projects, and a few chores.

At three in the morning on Monday, I turned in bed and felt like I was going to pee my pants. I rushed to the bathroom, just in time to feel the gush of water pouring out of me, and it wasn't my bladder at work.

My first thought: "Oh shit, my midwife is out of town." My second thought: "Is it okay to text the assistants at three in the morning to tell them my water broke?" I don't want to be rude, you know.

My husband, who normally works nights, happened to be home this particular morning and encouraged me to call them, which I did.

One of the assistants called me back. She told me to stay home and to check in with them when the contractions started and expect one of them to come over in a couple of hours. I texted my boss and told her I'd be working from home. She was very understanding. I worked for four hours, mainly wrapping up loose ends just in case this was my last shift before maternity leave.

Hubby finally installed the car seat that my folks had bought us and had been sitting in the living room for two months.

Around nine in the morning, the assistant came over and checked me. She said it could take hours before my labor began but suggested I rest and take it easy. I took the remainder of the day off and laid down for a nap next to my husband, who had gone back to sleep to be rested when the time came.

About an hour later, I woke up and realized my contractions had started. They felt like severe menstrual cramps, similar to those I experienced battling endometriosis in my early twenties. I thought, "This isn't too bad. I can handle this." The contractions became more regular and within the hour they started coming every five to seven minutes. Each one grew in intensity to the point I couldn't lay in bed anymore.

I got up and started doing some last minute stuff around the house—finishing packing my birthing center bag and throwing in some laundry—anything to mask the anxiety that came with each contraction.

As my contractions increased in intensity, all sorts of thoughts danced in my head, making me dizzy. What if I can't do this? What if I die? Worse, what if the baby dies? Oh, god, I'm going to end up in the hospital! I texted the midwife assistant and told her what was happening, minus the hurricane of fear brewing inside my gut. I didn't want to appear weak. She came over again.

When she knocked on my door, I was having a contraction leaning on the yoga ball, and couldn't even move to open it for her. That's how intense they were. Honestly, I don't know what early labor is because I went into active labor so quickly. Within minutes, the pain became unbearable. I got in the shower on my hand and knees. The hot water hitting my back seemed to take the edge off and let me breathe through the contractions. Water, blessed water. If I had water, I knew I could do this.

Soon afterward, the assistant came in and said it was time to go to the birthing center. Yes! That meant I was close. However, on the way there as we were pulling off the freeway, I had this crazy thought that I should tell Hubby to turn right instead of left and take me to the hospital. A strong contraction kept me from saying anything other than, "Oh hell, this hurts."

We arrived in the early afternoon. As soon as the tub was filled, I got in and relaxed into my labor. *Water goddess, here I come.* I let the water hold me, felt its warm embrace as I concentrated on opening my body to let the long-awaited child through. This is what I'd been waiting for. Unfortunately, it didn't last long.

I became cold as the water cooled. We added more hot, only to realize it was cold. Somehow they had run out of hot water for that particular room and tub. *Oh no, this couldn't be happening.*

To make matters worse, the room was cold, too. I shivered as I got out, which only made the contractions worse. By this point I couldn't take the pain. I became very vocal with each one. *Holy shit, it really did hurt.*

"Lower your voice," one of the assistants said, "and send that energy to your baby."

What? How does one send energy to a baby? I thought. *Furthermore, why would I want to send this pain to the baby?* She repeated this several times and told me to say "open" during the contractions. I did, but it didn't help with the pain or reduce the intensity. This was *not* the serene, natural, earthy childbirth I had anticipated. The longer it went, the deeper my fear festered.

At some point, the substitute midwife came in and introduced herself. She seemed pretty nice, but we didn't connect at all, mostly because I was in utter agony. To me, she felt like another assistant but not involved. Most of the time she stood in the shadows, letting the assistants do all the work and occasionally asked them how I was doing. She checked me after a while and said I was almost dilated and could start pushing soon.

By now it was dark outside, the fireplace was lit, the light turned down low, and candles burned everywhere. I looked around the room and thought this was the environment I wanted, but now that the time had arrived, none of it helped soothe my raging emotions. Boy was I ready to have this baby. I'd had enough of the pain. Baby needed to come and the sooner the better.

I pushed for what seemed like an eternity, but it was more like an hour or so. When the midwife checked me, I was fully dilated, but the baby hadn't moved down the birth canal. She suggested I walk around. I laughed. I could barely move; it hurt so much. The drugs at the hospital started to sound more appealing with each contraction.

For most of this, I didn't even know where my husband was. Turns out he'd left the room because he couldn't handle me screaming in pain and no one doing anything to ease it. That's what he told me later. He wanted to help so badly but didn't know how.

For natural pain relief they finally suggested I bounce on a yoga ball in the shower. And so I did. There I was, in a tiny slate-tiled shower stall, on the ball. Hot water cascading down my body, warm steam enveloping me; I was in my element at last. I drew strength from each droplet. The heat eased my pain, and I entered labor-land alone but fully empowered.

I felt like a goddess on her throne, finally able to focus my energy on pushing and opening rather than the pain of childbirth. Those forty-five magical minutes were exactly how I had envisioned my labor would be.

Unfortunately, when I came out of the shower and the midwife checked me, she said the baby still hadn't dropped. The baby also needed to turn her body and head slightly so she could move down the birth canal easier. Without the warm water therapy, the pain returned with a vengeance. The assistants tried different techniques to get the baby to turn, but the only thing that happened was more pain.

At this point I realized it could be hours before Baby came, and I had run out of steam. I was tired and had had enough. I remember thinking the whole natural birth thing was bullshit and pain-relieving drugs sounded really good. The epidural at the hospital called my name and I answered.

As requested, Hubby loaded me up in the car, and, with the accompaniment of the assistants, I was whisked to the hospital. I wept during the drive to the hospital, knowing this wasn't what I wanted but what I needed now. Yet a little voice whispered, "You should have listened to me when I suggested you turn right instead of left earlier. It would have saved you so much pain and suffering."

Within minutes of arrival, the anesthesiologist came in and administered an epidural. It took another ten minutes before I started feeling the effects. Relief! That doctor was the hero of the night, as far as I was concerned. If my legs hadn't been numb, I would have crawled out of my hospital bed and kissed him right then and there.

Now that I was at the hospital, my care was transferred to the midwives on duty at the hospital. The moment I met the night-shift midwife, I knew I should have been here the whole time. Every cell of my body knew this because I felt the tension melt away in that second. Between the labor nurses and the midwife, I knew I was in the presence of women who'd traveled down the road through birth-land. They understood my pain. The comfort this brought gave me hope that maybe I could get through the night and possibly actually have this baby.

They let me sleep for three hours. Blessed rest, finally. Oh, how my body and mind needed it. About three in the morning, the midwife started me on Pitocin, a labor-inducing medication. She started with a miniscule amount, measuring the pressure of my contractions with a catheter inserted into my uterus and adjusting the dosage accordingly. I had control of how much epidural medicine I received. This made me feel less guilty about my last-minute decision for medical interventions.

I was pretty numb but still could feel the pressure with each contraction. This allowed me to breathe through and focus on relaxing my pelvic muscles—a much better way to labor after the ordeal from the previous day. By eleven in the morning, it was time to push again.

To my amazement, they had me pushing in all sorts of positions. Hands and knees on the bed while the nurse and midwives held my knees and legs steady. Squatting at the foot of the bed, holding onto a bar. A whole variety of positions. I did not expect this from a hospital birth. In the hospital births I'd witnessed, the woman was strapped to the bed with her feet up in stirrups. That was the main reason I didn't want a hospital birth in the first place, but now I questioned all my decisions.

Had I made a mistake in going with an independent midwifery clinic rather than choosing the hospital midwifes? Doubt moved in. If I couldn't choose the right care that I needed, how would I be able to make decisions for the child I had yet to birth? Thankfully, I didn't have time to dwell on these things as all my focus fixed on pushing. *Please come out, Baby!*

After two hours of pushing, the midwife said the baby was stuck behind the pelvic bone. More than twenty-four hours had passed since my water broke, and she was concerned about the risk of infection, especially since I had had a urinary tract infection before going into the labor. She called in the surgeon to discuss my options. After everything I'd gone through, the thought of surgery freaked me out. He offered me a choice between vacuum and forceps or C-section. I wanted to avoid the latter at all costs so I chose the vacuum. He explained that while there were risks, because the baby had descended so low and just needed a little help turning her head and coming under the pelvic bone, she was a good candidate for this option.

The room filled with medical staff: three NICU nursing team members to resuscitate Baby in case she stopped breathing; my nurse; the midwife; the two midwife assistants from the birthing center; the baby's nurse; the surgeon; his assistant; and Hubby. Talk about a birthing "party." There I lay on the bed, propped up by pillows in all my naked glory, but I didn't give a rat's ass about modesty.

The only thing I cared about now was getting Baby out because I was tired. If I didn't do it now, the scary "C" loomed over me like a haggard witch with long, grubby fingers waiting to snatch my baby girl from me. I could almost hear her cackles. By golly, I wasn't going let her win after all my hard work. At least not if there was a chance I could still deliver vaginally.

Ready, set, go! Let's do this thing. I started to push again on the doctor's cue. With each push, he suctioned the baby's head down a little more. On each contraction, he coached me on where to push and for how long. I didn't think I had any more strength left, but the doctor encouraged me and somehow I found a few extra ounces of hidden energy. Like an angel sent from the heavenly realms, he guided me through the last leg of my wild birthing journey. Four contractions and my baby girl came out.

When I saw the slimy, bloody, little human lying in his hands between my legs, my heart almost stopped.

I'd spent most of my life not wanting kids. Sure, I loved children—other people's offspring, that is—but I'd never felt the urge to procreate myself. I had spent my entire adult life avoiding getting pregnant. I also didn't think I would ever marry either. I was pretty happy living my own life.

Then I met my husband. Everything changed. I knew I could be a wife to him and bear his children within the first week we met. For someone independent like me, that said something about the awesomeness of the man who's my partner, best friend, soul mate, lover, and spouse. And now we finally had our daughter.

The nurse put my baby on my chest. I held her close and kissed her wet, gooey, little head of black hair. She was mine. All mine. I'd done it. I'd carried her for nine months, felt her kicks, talked to her, wondered what she'd look like, and now she was here in my arms. They took her away for a few moments to do her assessments and vitals but brought her right back. Skin to skin, she lay on my chest. One slow wiggle at a time, she made her way to my breast. Within twenty minutes she found my left nipple and latched on naturally.

While I bonded with my daughter—which was more like "let the shock sink in" that I was a mother now—the surgeon sewed up my perineum. I had a third-degree tear. I didn't feel it because of the epidural. I didn't care, though, because I'd avoided a C-section and I had Baby vaginally. I owed that man a debt of gratitude for helping me bring my little angel into the world, even if she did have a cone-head thing going on from the vacuum extraction.

Once the drugs wore off, I did care about my condition. I couldn't sit, much less walk, because of the stitches and my bruised tail bone. The baby's head had done a number on my pelvic area. It felt like someone had taken a bat and machete down there. Oh, my! And trying to pee was like spraying acid on a raw wound.

I questioned what the hell I had been thinking, and, in my dark state of mind, I wondered if a C-section might have been a better option. *Who thinks that?* I mentally slapped myself. For once, I understood why some women chose that route, and I knew I would never ever judge them. It hurt just to pass gas, and I freaked out about when the time came to poop. The midwife put me on stool softeners which helped. Ice packs and good ol' narcotics helped ease the discomfort.

Oh, and did I mention sore nipples? Yes, breastfeeding is amazing and great for bonding and the baby's health, but OH. MY. GOD. OUCH!!! Yet it didn't matter to me because I was determined to breastfeed my daughter even though my nipples felt on fire every time she nursed.

Unfortunately, breastfeeding did not come easy. I had lactation specialists come in every day during my hospital stay, sometimes several times during the day, showing me how to get Baby to latch on and encouraging me to pump after every feeding. So not only was I waking up every two hours to feed her, I had to spend another fifteen minutes pumping a few extra drops of colostrum and then clean the equipment so it would be ready for the next use. It felt pointless to try to sleep in between feedings.

Shortly after I delivered, I spiked a fever. The midwife put me and the baby on antibiotics. I wanted to cry every time I looked at the clean diaper wrapped around her right arm to protect the IV line. The invisible words written all over the white material flashed at me: "You did this because you chose to come to the hospital. Because you were too weak to have her naturally."

The second day at the hospital, Baby became jaundiced. She spent twelve hours under bilirubin lights—the longest day ever while we were in the hospital. The sight of the machine next to my hospital bed was just another slap in the face for my failure.

The third day, when we should have been going home, our blood work revealed I was fine but my daughter's white blood cell count had gone up. The good news was that her immune system worked; the bad news was that we needed to stay for another two days so she could complete her antibiotic regime, even though her blood cultures came back negative. The pediatrician said it was better to keep her two more days than to go home and risk having her become ill. A second hospitalization would be worse. I completely agreed.

We were transferred to the Children's Hospital next door. It felt silly having NICU nurses taking care of my baby just to have antibiotics administered when other babies were there with much more serious problems. At least they had one easy patient.

The following day, her IV became infiltrated and a new one had to be put in. Hubby had gone home to get a few things, and I didn't have the courage to watch the procedure alone. The medical staff took her into another room. The whole time, I felt like the worst mother for not having the strength to be there for my baby, but I simply couldn't watch unless they were ready to put an IV in me and give me a sedative. A half hour later, the nurse told me they are going to get the IV specialist. Another half hour passed. The nurse said they couldn't get the IV in, and they were calling the care flight nurse because she was the best. Well, she couldn't do it either. Finally they talked to the doctor to see what other options were available for administering the antibiotics. It turned out she only needed three intramuscular shots and that was it.

The nurse felt awful, but I felt worse when I saw all of the Band-Aids covering Baby's body. If I learned anything from the experience, it was that my little girl is one tough cookie and stubborn as a bull, kind of like her mama used to be. If only I had been stubborn enough to birth her at the center and avoid all of this.

The next morning her blood test showed everything was normal, and we were allowed to go home. Bringing home Baby was the best gift imaginable. We received the highest-rated care possible in the hospital. All of the nurses, midwives, lactation specialist, and doctors rocked. But there was nothing like being home. Little did I know the hardest part hadn't even begun.

Read more here (www.amazon.com).

Made in the USA
Middletown, DE
19 May 2015